THE PEGAN DIET

A Comprehensive Guide to Paleo
and Vegan Fusion for Optimal
Health and Weight Loss

Dr. Raymond F. Bernard

TABLE OF CONTENTS

CHAPTER 1

Introduction to the Pegan Diet

In this first chapter, we delve into the fascinating world of the Pegan diet. Let's break down this concept in plain human language, exploring its origins, principles, and why it has captured the attention of health-conscious individuals around the world.

What is the Pegan Diet?

The Pegan diet might sound like a quirky name, but it represents a thoughtful approach to nutrition that combines principles from two popular diets: Paleo and Vegan. To understand the Pegan diet, we need to first grasp the basics of its parent diets.

Paleo Diet: The Paleo diet, short for Paleolithic diet, takes inspiration from the eating habits of our ancient ancestors. It emphasizes whole, unprocessed foods like lean meats, fish, fruits, vegetables, nuts, and seeds. The key idea is to exclude modern processed foods and grains, as they weren't part of our ancestors' diets.

Vegan Diet: On the other end of the spectrum, we have the Vegan diet, which excludes all animal products. It's a plant-based diet that focuses on fruits, vegetables, grains, legumes, nuts, and seeds. Veganism is often chosen for ethical, environmental, and health reasons.

The Birth of Peganism: The Pegan diet emerged as a middle ground between these two diets. It acknowledges that while our ancestors did consume animal products, our modern food system is fraught with issues like factory farming and overconsumption of meat. The Pegan diet encourages a strong focus on plant-based foods, but it doesn't entirely eliminate high-quality animal products. It promotes the consumption of sustainably sourced, grass-fed meats and wild-caught fish.

The Core Principles of Pegan

Now, let's explore the principles that form the core of the Pegan diet:

1. **Plant-Based Emphasis**: The Pegan diet centers around plant foods. This

means a significant portion of your plate should be filled with colorful fruits and vegetables. They provide essential vitamins, minerals, and fiber.

2. **Healthy Fats**: It welcomes the consumption of healthy fats from sources like avocados, nuts, seeds, and olive oil. These fats are associated with heart health and overall well-being.

3. **Limited Processed Foods**: Just like the Paleo diet, Pegan discourages processed foods. Highly processed items are often

laden with unhealthy additives, preservatives, and excessive sugar.

4. **Quality Protein**: While Pegan doesn't eliminate animal products, it places great importance on the quality of these sources. Grass-fed meats, pasture-raised poultry, and wild-caught fish are favored over conventionally raised meats.

5. **Gluten and Dairy Awareness**: Pegan diets tend to minimize or eliminate gluten and dairy. Many people are sensitive to these substances, and

avoiding them can improve digestive health.

6. **Balanced Macronutrients**: A balanced intake of macronutrients (carbohydrates, proteins, and fats) is key. The idea is to avoid extreme restrictions on any one nutrient.

7. **Mindful Eating**: Pegan emphasizes the importance of mindful eating. This means paying attention to your body's hunger and fullness cues, eating slowly, and savoring each bite.

8. **Sustainability**:

Sustainability is a big focus. It encourages choices that are not only healthy for our bodies but also for the planet. This includes supporting local and organic agriculture and reducing food waste.

Why Peganism Matters

You might wonder, with so many diets out there, why should you care about the Pegan diet? Well, there are several reasons why this diet has gained traction and is worth exploring:

Health Benefits: The Pegan diet combines the best of both worlds - the health benefits of a plant-based diet with the nutrients found in high-quality animal products. Research suggests that this balance can be beneficial for heart health, weight management, and overall well-being.

Digestive Health: By limiting processed foods, gluten, and dairy, the Pegan diet can be gentler on your digestive system. Many people report improved gut health and reduced digestive discomfort when following this approach.

Ethical Considerations: If you're concerned about the ethical treatment of animals and the environmental impact of your food choices, Peganism provides a framework for making conscious choices that align with these values.

Sustainability: As our world grapples with sustainability challenges, the Pegan diet promotes a more sustainable way of eating. By reducing reliance on resource-intensive animal agriculture and favoring plant-based foods, it contributes to a healthier planet.

Food Quality Matters: Peganism underscores the importance of food quality. It encourages you to think not just about what you eat but also where it comes from. This can lead to a deeper connection with your food and a greater appreciation for the farmers and producers behind it.

A Holistic Approach: Unlike many diets that focus solely on weight loss or a specific health outcome, the Pegan diet takes a holistic approach to health. It recognizes that our well-being is interconnected with the health of our planet and the ethical treatment of animals.

Closing Thoughts

In Chapter 1, we've laid the foundation for understanding the Pegan diet. It's a dietary approach that seeks balance, sustainability, and health. It's not about rigid rules or extreme restrictions; rather, it's a flexible and mindful way of eating that can be tailored to your individual preferences and values.

As we continue through this book, we'll dive deeper into the science behind Pegan, practical tips for adopting this diet, its impact on health, ethical considerations, and the future trends that might shape the Pegan landscape. So, if you're curious about exploring a diet that combines the wisdom of our ancestors with the needs of our modern world, keep reading. The journey into the Pegan diet has only just begun.

CHAPTER 2

The Science Behind Pegan

Welcome to Chapter 2 of our exploration of the Pegan diet. In this chapter, we're going to dive deep into the scientific principles that underpin the Pegan diet. You'll discover why Peganism isn't just another dietary trend but is rooted in evidence-based reasoning. So, let's unpack the science in simple human language.

Understanding the Basics of Pegan Science

Before we dive into the specifics, it's essential to grasp the fundamental scientific ideas that guide the Pegan diet.

1. **Nutrient Density**: Peganism places a strong emphasis on nutrient-dense foods. These are foods that are packed with vitamins, minerals, and other essential nutrients per calorie. The goal is to get the most nutrition out of every bite you take.

2. **Inflammation**: Chronic inflammation is increasingly recognized as a root cause of

many diseases, from heart disease to diabetes. The Pegan diet is designed to reduce inflammation through food choices.

3. **Balanced Macronutrients**: While Pegan leans towards plant-based foods, it doesn't exclude any macronutrient category. It encourages a balanced intake of carbohydrates, proteins, and fats, recognizing that each plays a unique role in our health.

Now, let's delve into some of the scientific principles that make Peganism compelling:

Plant-Based Nutrients: Peganism's strong focus on plant-based foods isn't just a matter of preference; it's backed by substantial scientific evidence. Research consistently shows that plant-rich diets are associated with reduced risk of chronic diseases such as heart disease, stroke, and certain cancers. The fiber, antioxidants, and phytochemicals found in fruits and vegetables play a vital role in promoting health.

Healthy Fats: Another key aspect of Peganism is the inclusion of healthy fats like those from avocados, nuts, and olive oil. Science supports this choice. These fats are rich in monounsaturated and polyunsaturated fats, which are known to have a positive impact on heart health. They can help lower bad cholesterol levels and reduce the risk of heart disease.

Limited Processed Foods: The Pegan diet's avoidance of processed foods aligns with scientific consensus. Highly processed foods are often high in added sugars, unhealthy fats, and sodium. Numerous studies link the consumption of these foods to obesity, type 2 diabetes, and cardiovascular disease.

Quality Protein: While Peganism doesn't exclude animal products, it does emphasize the quality of these sources. Grass-fed meats and wild-caught fish, for instance, have a different nutrient profile than conventionally raised counterparts. They tend to be leaner and contain higher levels of beneficial omega-3 fatty acids. Science supports the idea that these higher quality animal products can contribute positively to health.

Gluten and Dairy Awareness: Peganism's cautious approach to gluten and dairy is rooted in scientific understanding. Some people are sensitive to gluten, a protein found in wheat, barley, and rye, leading to conditions like celiac disease or non-celiac gluten sensitivity. Similarly, lactose intolerance is common, making dairy problematic for many individuals.

Balanced Macronutrients: The Pegan diet's emphasis on balanced macronutrients isn't just a whim.

Carbohydrates, proteins, and fats each play vital roles in our bodies. Carbs provide energy, proteins are the building blocks of our cells, and fats are essential for various bodily functions, including brain health. By promoting a balance, Peganism aims to provide your body with all the nutrients it needs for optimal functioning.

Inflammation Reduction: Chronic inflammation is a hot topic in scientific research. It's linked to a wide range of health issues, from cardiovascular disease to autoimmune conditions. The Pegan diet's anti-inflammatory approach, with its focus on whole, unprocessed foods and omega-3-rich fats, aligns with strategies for reducing inflammation.

The Role of Gut Health: Emerging research suggests that the health of our gut microbiome, the trillions of microorganisms in our digestive system, has a profound impact on overall health. Peganism, with its emphasis on fiber-rich foods like fruits and vegetables, can support a diverse and healthy gut microbiome.

Ethical and Environmental Considerations: While not

purely scientific, the ethical and environmental aspects of the Pegan diet are firmly grounded in facts. Factory farming, for instance, is known to have detrimental effects on animal welfare, and it contributes significantly to greenhouse gas emissions. By advocating for sustainably sourced animal products and reduced meat consumption, Peganism aligns with environmental and ethical concerns.

Personalization and Evidence-Based Practice: It's important to note that the Pegan diet, like any dietary approach, isn't a one-size-fits-all solution. The science behind Peganism supports the idea that individual needs and preferences should be taken into account. Personalization is a key element of the Pegan diet, allowing people to tailor it to their unique health goals and lifestyles.

In summary, the science behind the Pegan diet is firmly grounded in established nutritional principles. It combines the health benefits of plant-based eating with the nutritional advantages of high-quality animal products. It addresses concerns related to inflammation, processed foods, and the ethical and environmental impacts of dietary choices.

As you progress through this book, you'll gain a deeper understanding of how to apply these scientific principles in your daily life. We'll explore practical tips, meal planning, and real-world success stories that showcase the tangible health benefits of adopting a Pegan approach to eating. So, stay tuned for the practical wisdom that lies ahead in the chapters to come.

CHAPTER 3

The Pegan Diet in Practice

Welcome to Chapter 3, where we're going to roll up our sleeves and get practical about the Pegan diet. This chapter is all about taking those core principles we discussed earlier and translating them into actionable steps for your everyday life. So, let's dive in and explore how to put the Pegan diet into practice without stress or confusion.

Getting Started with the Pegan Diet

So, you're intrigued by the idea of the Pegan diet, but where do you begin? Here's a step-by-step guide to help you embark on your Pegan journey:

1. Learn the Basics: Review the core principles of the Pegan diet. Remember, it's about emphasizing plant-based foods, choosing high-quality proteins, and avoiding processed junk.

2. Clean Out Your Pantry: Take stock of your kitchen. Donate or discard heavily processed foods, sugary snacks, and foods containing unhealthy trans fats.

3. Plan Your Meals: Planning is your ally. Sketch out a weekly meal plan that includes a variety of colorful vegetables, fruits, lean proteins, nuts, seeds, and healthy fats.

4. Gradual Changes: Transitioning to a new way of eating can be daunting. Consider making gradual changes to give your taste buds and digestion time to adjust.

5. Shop Smart: Make a grocery list based on your meal plan.

Focus on the perimeter of the store where you'll find fresh produce, lean proteins, and whole grains.

6. Prep Ahead: Spend some time prepping ingredients over the weekend. Wash and chop vegetables, cook grains, and marinate proteins. This can save you time during busy weekdays.

7. Experiment and Explore: Don't be afraid to try new foods and recipes. Peganism opens up a world of culinary exploration, so get creative in the kitchen.

8. Stay Hydrated: Water is essential. Stay hydrated throughout the day to support digestion and overall well-being.

Practical Tips for Meal Planning

Meal planning is a cornerstone of the Pegan diet. Here's how to create balanced and satisfying meals:

1. The Pegan Plate: Visualize your plate as divided into three sections: 50% colorful vegetables, 25% lean protein, and 25% healthy fats and complex carbs.

2. Breakfast Inspiration: Opt for a nutrient-packed smoothie with leafy greens, berries, a scoop of protein powder, and a tablespoon of almond butter.

3. Lunch Ideas: Create a big salad with mixed greens, grilled chicken, avocado slices, roasted vegetables, and a drizzle of olive oil and lemon juice.

4. Dinner Delights: Enjoy a serving of baked salmon with quinoa and a side of steamed broccoli. Top it off with a handful of crushed nuts for crunch.

5. Snacking Smart: Keep snacks like carrot sticks, cucumber slices, and a handful of mixed nuts on hand for when hunger strikes between meals.

6. Hydration Heroes: Herbal teas, infused water with citrus slices, and coconut water are great options for staying hydrated.

Overcoming Challenges and Staying Consistent

The path to adopting the Pegan diet isn't always smooth, but with a few strategies, you can overcome common challenges:

1. Social Situations: Eating out or attending social events? Look for options that align with Pegan principles. Most restaurants offer salads with protein options.

2. Cravings: If you're craving something sweet, opt for a piece of fruit or a small handful of berries. They provide natural sweetness along with fiber and nutrients.

3. Traveling: Pack snacks like trail mix, cut vegetables, and fruit to have healthy options on hand during your journey.

4. Busy Schedule: Batch cooking can be a lifesaver. Cook larger portions and store leftovers for quick and convenient meals.

5. Finding Support: Join online communities or forums of fellow Pegans for recipe ideas, tips, and support.

6. Flexibility: Remember that flexibility is key. If you're at a social gathering and there's a delicious non-Pegan dish, it's okay to enjoy it occasionally without guilt.

Navigating Pegan for Different Lifestyles

The beauty of the Pegan diet is its flexibility. It can be tailored to different dietary preferences and needs:

1. **Vegan Pegans**: Focus on plant-based proteins like lentils, beans, tofu, and tempeh. Load up on vegetables and healthy fats from nuts, seeds, and avocados.

2. **Omnivore Pegans**: Incorporate high-quality animal products such as grass-fed beef, free-range poultry, and wild-caught fish into your meals.

3. **Vegetarian Pegans**: Emphasize plant-based proteins like beans, legumes, quinoa, and eggs. Make sure to include a

variety of colorful vegetables and whole grains.

4. Picky Eaters: If you're selective about certain foods, focus on the ones you enjoy while keeping the Pegan principles in mind. Gradually introduce new foods to expand your palate.

5. Family-Friendly Peganism: Transitioning your family to a Pegan-style diet might require a gradual approach. Involve them in meal planning and cooking to make it a shared experience.

In Conclusion

Chapter 3 has provided you with a practical roadmap to bring the Pegan diet into your daily life. By starting small, planning your meals, and staying adaptable, you'll find that adopting Pegan principles becomes second nature. The journey to better health, ethical eating, and a more sustainable lifestyle starts with these simple steps.

As you continue reading this book, we'll delve into the health benefits of the Pegan diet, strategies to maintain long-term success, and even explore some delicious Pegan-friendly recipes to tantalize your taste buds. So, get ready to savor the journey as you transform your eating habits and embrace the Pegan way of life.

CHAPTER 4

Pegan Plate - Creating Balanced Meals

Welcome to Chapter 4, where we'll unravel the art of constructing balanced and satisfying meals following the Pegan diet principles. In this chapter, we'll break down the Pegan Plate concept, share sample meal plans, and provide you with ideas to ignite your culinary creativity. Let's embark on a delicious journey into the world of Pegan meal creation.

The Pegan Plate: A Blueprint for Balance

At the heart of the Pegan diet is the concept of the Pegan Plate. Think of it as a visual guide to help you craft nutritious and satisfying meals. Here's the breakdown:

1. **50% Colorful Vegetables**: Half of your plate should be filled with a vibrant array of vegetables. Aim for a variety of colors to ensure you're getting a broad spectrum of nutrients. Leafy greens, bell peppers, carrots, broccoli, and beets are just a few examples.

2. **25% Lean Protein**: A quarter of your plate is devoted to protein. Lean protein sources can include grilled chicken, turkey, tofu, tempeh, legumes, or fish like salmon or trout. These options are rich in essential amino acids to support your body's growth and repair.

3. **25% Healthy Fats and Complex Carbohydrates**: The remaining quarter is split between healthy fats and complex carbohydrates. Healthy fats can come from avocado, nuts, seeds, or olive oil. Complex carbohydrates

are found in foods like quinoa, sweet potatoes, and whole grains such as brown rice.

Sample Meal Plans for Different Preferences

To give you a practical sense of how the Pegan Plate can translate into your meals, here are three sample meal plans tailored to different dietary preferences:

1. Vegan Pegan Meal Plan:

- **Breakfast**: A smoothie with kale, banana, almond butter, chia seeds, and almond milk.

- **Lunch**: A colorful salad with mixed greens, chickpeas, cherry tomatoes, cucumber, and tahini dressing.

- **Dinner**: Stir-fried tofu with broccoli, bell peppers, and a ginger-soy sauce, served over quinoa.

- **Snack**: Sliced avocado on whole-grain toast with a sprinkle of nutritional yeast.

2. **Omnivore Pegan Meal Plan**:

- **Breakfast**: Scrambled eggs with spinach and tomatoes, and a side of sliced avocado.

- **Lunch**: A salad with mixed greens, grilled chicken, strawberries, and a balsamic vinaigrette.

- **Dinner**: Baked salmon with asparagus and a side of quinoa cooked in vegetable broth.

- **Snack**: A handful of mixed nuts and a piece of fruit.

3. Vegetarian Pegan Meal Plan:

- **Breakfast**: Greek yogurt topped with berries, almonds, and a drizzle of honey.

- **Lunch**: A bowl of lentil soup with a side of roasted Brussels sprouts.
- **Dinner**: Stuffed bell peppers with a mixture of quinoa, black beans, corn, and diced tomatoes.
- **Snack**: Sliced cucumber and carrot sticks with hummus.

These meal plans offer a glimpse into the variety and flexibility of the Pegan diet. While they provide structure, remember that the Pegan Plate is a guide, not a rigid rule. Feel free to mix and match ingredients to suit your taste and dietary needs.

Culinary Creativity in Pegan Cooking

One of the joys of following the Pegan diet is the opportunity to get creative in the kitchen. Here are some ideas to spark your culinary imagination:

1. Pegan Bowls: Create colorful bowls with a base of quinoa or cauliflower rice, topped with an assortment of roasted and raw vegetables, a protein source, and a flavorful sauce.

2. Pegan Stir-Fries: Stir-fry is a versatile Pegan-friendly dish. Combine tofu, tempeh, or lean meat with an array of vegetables, and season with Pegan-approved sauces like tamari or coconut aminos.

3. Veggie-Centric Pasta: Replace traditional pasta with spiralized zucchini or sweet potato noodles. Top them with a Pegan-friendly tomato or pesto sauce and add your choice of protein.

4. Power-Packed Salads: Elevate your salads with ingredients like roasted beets, walnuts, pomegranate seeds, and citrus segments. Experiment with different greens, and don't forget a drizzle of olive oil and lemon juice.

5. Pegan Snacking: Prepare Pegan-friendly snacks like kale chips, trail mix with nuts and seeds, or apple slices with almond butter.

6. Pegan Breakfasts: Breakfast can be a time to load up on veggies. Try omelets filled with sautéed spinach, mushrooms, and bell peppers, or a sweet potato hash with eggs.

Pegan Meal Planning and Prep

Effective meal planning and preparation can be your Pegan

diet allies. Here's how to streamline these processes:

1. Weekly Meal Planning: Dedicate time each week to plan your meals. This helps you create a balanced grocery list and ensures you have the ingredients you need.

2. Batch Cooking: Cook larger batches of grains, proteins, and roasted vegetables to use in multiple meals throughout the week. It saves time and reduces daily cooking stress.

3. Stock Up on Staples: Keep Pegan-friendly staples in your pantry, such as canned beans, whole grains, nuts, and seeds. These items provide a solid foundation for your meals.

4. Use Leftovers Wisely: Be creative with leftovers. Turn last night's roasted vegetables into a frittata or add cooked quinoa to a salad for extra substance.

5. Freeze Ahead: Prepare extra portions of soups, stews, or casseroles and freeze them in single servings for future quick and healthy meals.

Practical Tips for Eating Out Pegan-Style

Eating out while following the Pegan diet can be enjoyable and stress-free with these tips:

1. Plan Ahead: Check the restaurant's menu online beforehand to identify Pegan-friendly options.

2. Customization: Don't hesitate to ask for substitutions or alterations to make a dish Pegan-friendly. For example, request extra vegetables or avocado in your salad.

3. Dressing on the Side: Ask for salad dressings and sauces on the side so you can control how much you use.

4. Protein Choices: Look for dishes with lean protein sources, such as grilled chicken or fish, or plant-based options like tofu.

5. Be Mindful: Pay attention to portion sizes. Restaurant portions can be larger than what you'd typically eat at home.

6. Savor the Moment: Enjoy your dining experience and the social aspect of eating out. Focus on the company, not just the food.

In Conclusion

Chapter 4 has unraveled the art of creating balanced and delicious meals following the Pegan diet principles. Whether you're a vegan, an omnivore, or somewhere in between, the Pegan Plate offers a flexible framework for constructing nourishing and satisfying dishes.

As you continue reading this book, you'll explore the health benefits of the Pegan diet, including its impact on weight management and gut health. You'll also discover the ethical and sustainable aspects of Peganism, gaining a holistic understanding of how this dietary approach can positively influence your well-being and the world around you. So, get ready to savor the flavors and embrace the Pegan way of eating with enthusiasm.

CHAPTER 5

Pegan Diet and Health

Welcome to Chapter 5, where we delve into the significant impact of the Pegan diet on your health. The Pegan diet isn't just about what you eat; it's about how it can transform your well-being. In this chapter, we'll explore the health benefits associated with the Pegan diet, its role in weight management, and its effects on gut health. So, let's dive into the science and practical aspects of Peganism for a healthier you.

Unlocking the Health Benefits of the Pegan Diet

The Pegan diet's core principles - emphasizing plant-based foods, healthy fats, and high-quality protein sources while minimizing processed foods - have been linked to several health benefits:

1. **Heart Health**: The Pegan diet's focus on healthy fats, like those from avocados and nuts, along with lean protein sources, can promote heart health. These components can help lower LDL

(bad) cholesterol levels and reduce the risk of heart disease.

2. Weight Management: The Pegan diet's nutrient-dense approach can be beneficial for weight management. By filling your plate with vegetables and quality proteins, you naturally reduce calorie-dense processed foods, which can help with weight loss or maintenance.

3. Blood Sugar Control: The Pegan diet's emphasis on whole, unprocessed foods can help stabilize blood sugar levels. It includes complex carbohydrates from sources like sweet potatoes and whole grains, which are digested more slowly, preventing rapid spikes in blood sugar.

4. Improved Digestion: Peganism, with its fiber-rich vegetables and fruits, supports digestive health. Adequate fiber intake can aid in regular bowel movements and contribute to a healthy gut microbiome.

5. Reduced Inflammation: Chronic inflammation is a contributing factor to various health issues, including heart disease and autoimmune conditions. The Pegan diet's anti-inflammatory components, such as omega-3 fatty acids from fish and antioxidants from fruits and vegetables, can help reduce inflammation.

6. Better Nutrient Intake: By focusing on nutrient-dense foods, the Pegan diet ensures you get a wide range of vitamins, minerals, and antioxidants essential for overall health.

7. Balanced Macronutrients: The Pegan diet promotes a balanced intake of macronutrients, including carbohydrates, proteins, and fats. This balance can help regulate energy levels and support various bodily functions.

The Pegan Diet and Weight Management

Weight management is a significant concern for many, and the Pegan diet can be a valuable tool in achieving and maintaining a healthy weight. Here's how it can help:

1. **Satiety**: The Pegan diet's emphasis on fiber-rich vegetables and fruits, combined with quality proteins and fats, can increase feelings of fullness and reduce overeating.

2. **Reduced Calorie-Dense Foods**: By limiting processed and

calorie-dense foods, the Pegan diet naturally reduces calorie intake, which can lead to weight loss.

3. Balanced Blood Sugar: Stable blood sugar levels are crucial for weight management. The Pegan diet's avoidance of refined sugars and emphasis on complex carbohydrates can help regulate blood sugar and reduce cravings.

4. Healthy Fats: Including healthy fats like avocados and nuts in the diet can help you feel satisfied and reduce the desire for high-calorie, low-nutrient snacks.

5. Nutrient Density: Even when reducing calorie intake, the Pegan diet ensures you receive essential nutrients, which is crucial for maintaining health while losing weight.

Gut Health and the Pegan Diet

Emerging research has highlighted the critical role of the gut microbiome in overall health. The Pegan diet can positively influence gut health in several ways:

1. Fiber-Rich Foods: The Pegan diet includes an abundance of fiber from vegetables, fruits, and whole grains. Fiber serves as food for beneficial gut bacteria, promoting a diverse and healthy microbiome.

2. Reduced Processed Foods: Processed foods, often lacking fiber and essential nutrients, can negatively impact the gut microbiome. By minimizing these foods, the Pegan diet supports a healthier gut.

3. Plant Diversity: Consuming a variety of plant-based foods provides different types of fiber and compounds that nourish a broader range of gut bacteria.

4. Prebiotics and Probiotics: Some Pegan-friendly foods, like fermented vegetables and yogurt (if dairy is included), can provide probiotics that introduce beneficial bacteria to the gut. Additionally, the fiber-rich nature of the diet acts as a prebiotic, feeding existing gut bacteria.

5. Reduced Inflammation: Chronic inflammation can disrupt the gut microbiome. The anti-inflammatory components of the Pegan diet may help create a more favorable environment for beneficial gut bacteria.

Practical Tips for Optimal Health on the Pegan Diet

To maximize the health benefits of the Pegan diet, consider these practical tips:

1. Variety is Key: Aim for a wide variety of vegetables, fruits, and plant-based foods to ensure you receive a broad spectrum of nutrients and promote a diverse gut microbiome.

2. Mindful Eating: Pay attention to your body's hunger and fullness cues. Eating slowly and savoring your food can help prevent overeating.

3. Hydration: Stay adequately hydrated by drinking water throughout the day. Proper hydration supports digestion and overall health.

4. Quality Matters: When choosing animal products, prioritize high-quality, sustainably sourced options. Grass-fed meats and wild-caught fish are examples.

5. Watch Portion Sizes: While nutrient-dense, Pegan-friendly foods can still contribute calories. Be mindful of portion sizes to maintain a healthy weight.

6. Experiment and Enjoy: Don't be afraid to experiment with new recipes and ingredients. Embrace the joy of cooking and savoring delicious, healthful meals.

Peganism Beyond Health: A Holistic Approach

The Pegan diet's impact extends beyond personal health. It embodies a holistic approach that encompasses ethical and environmental considerations:

1. Ethical Eating: By favoring sustainably sourced animal products and reducing meat consumption, the Pegan diet aligns with ethical concerns about animal welfare.

2. Sustainability: Peganism supports a more sustainable food system by reducing reliance on resource-intensive animal agriculture and promoting locally sourced, seasonal produce.

3. Connection to Food: Embracing the Pegan diet often means a deeper connection to the food you eat. Understanding where your food comes from and how it's produced can lead to more conscious and responsible choices.

Closing Thoughts

Chapter 5 has illuminated the significant impact of the Pegan diet on health, including its role in weight management and gut health. This dietary approach isn't just about what you eat; it's a holistic way of nourishing your body and aligning your food choices with ethical and environmental values.

As you continue reading this book, you'll delve deeper into the practical aspects of Peganism, from recipes to meal planning strategies. You'll also explore the sustainability and ethical considerations associated with the Pegan diet, gaining a well-rounded understanding of how this dietary approach can benefit not only your health but also the world around you. So, get ready to continue your journey towards optimal health and conscious eating with the Pegan diet as your guide.

CHAPTER 6

Sustainable and Ethical Eating with the Pegan Diet

Welcome to Chapter 6, where we delve into the ethical and sustainable aspects of the Pegan diet. Beyond its impact on personal health, the Pegan diet aligns with values related to animal welfare, environmental sustainability, and responsible food choices. In this chapter, we'll explore how the Pegan diet promotes ethical and sustainable eating, its contribution to reducing food waste, and its potential to shape a more responsible food system.

Peganism and Ethical Eating

Ethical eating is a cornerstone of the Pegan diet. It recognizes the ethical dilemmas associated with modern food production and offers a path to more conscientious choices:

1. **Animal Welfare**: Peganism encourages the consumption of high-quality, sustainably sourced animal products, such as grass-fed meats and wild-caught fish. These

choices often come from more humane and ethical farming practices.

2. Reducing Animal Suffering: By opting for animal products from sources that prioritize animal welfare, Pegans contribute to reducing the suffering of animals raised in less humane conditions.

3. Supporting Sustainable Farming: Choosing locally sourced and sustainably raised animal products helps support farmers and producers who prioritize ethical and environmentally responsible practices.

4. Reducing Factory Farming: Peganism's emphasis on reducing meat consumption can contribute to a decrease in the demand for factory-farmed animal products, which are often associated with poor animal welfare conditions.

5. Mindful Eating: Pegans are encouraged to be mindful of their food choices, considering the ethical implications of their diet. This mindfulness can lead to more responsible choices in alignment with personal values.

Sustainability and the Pegan Diet

Sustainability is another key pillar of the Pegan diet. It addresses the environmental concerns associated with modern food production and distribution:

1. **Sustainable Agriculture**: The Pegan diet promotes a diet rich in plant-based foods, which tend to have a lower environmental footprint compared to animal agriculture. This shift can contribute to more sustainable land use and reduced resource consumption.

2. Reducing Greenhouse Gas Emissions: Factory farming is a significant contributor to greenhouse gas emissions. By choosing sustainably sourced animal products or reducing meat consumption, Pegans can help mitigate these emissions.

3. Supporting Local Farmers: Embracing locally sourced and seasonal produce can support local farmers and reduce the carbon footprint associated with long-distance transportation of food.

4. Decreasing Food Waste: The Pegan diet's emphasis on mindful eating and reduced processed foods can help reduce food waste, a significant sustainability concern. Pegans are encouraged to use ingredients fully and repurpose leftovers creatively.

5. Encouraging Responsible Fishing: When Pegans choose fish, they often prioritize wild-caught options. This choice supports responsible fishing practices that aim to maintain healthy ocean ecosystems.

6. Sustainable Packaging: Pegans often gravitate toward minimally processed foods with simple packaging, which can reduce waste and contribute to a more sustainable food system.

Reducing Food Waste with Peganism

Food waste is a global issue with significant ethical and environmental consequences. The Pegan diet can play a role in addressing this problem:

1. Mindful Meal Planning: Pegans often plan their meals in advance, reducing the likelihood of buying excess food that may go to waste.

2. Using Leftovers Creatively: Leftovers are repurposed into new meals, reducing food waste. For example, roasted vegetables can become a frittata, and cooked grains can be added to salads.

3. Whole Food Emphasis: The Pegan diet encourages the use of whole, unprocessed foods. These foods often have a longer shelf life and can be used more efficiently in cooking.

4. Composting: Pegans who have access to composting facilities can reduce food waste by composting scraps, contributing to healthier soil and less waste in landfills.

5. Responsible Shopping: Pegans are mindful shoppers, buying what they need and avoiding excessive purchases that might lead to food spoilage.

A Path to Responsible Food Choices

The Pegan diet offers a clear path to responsible and ethical food choices. Whether it's selecting humanely raised animal products, supporting local and sustainable agriculture, or reducing food waste, Pegans have a framework to align their eating habits with values of compassion and environmental responsibility.

Peganism and Sustainable Agriculture

Sustainable agriculture practices are integral to the Pegan diet's ethos:

1. **Organic Choices**: Many Pegans choose organic produce to minimize exposure to pesticides and support farming practices that prioritize soil health.

2. **Local and Seasonal Eating**: Pegans often prioritize local and seasonal produce. This reduces the carbon footprint associated with food transportation and supports regional agriculture.

3. Regenerative Farming: Some Pegans go a step further by supporting regenerative farming practices, which aim to restore and cnhance soil health while sequestering carbon.

4. Reduced Meat Consumption: By reducing meat consumption, Pegans contribute to a more sustainable food system. Factory farming, a common source of meat, is known for its resource-intensive practices and environmental impact.

Peganism and Responsible Fishing

The Pegan diet's focus on fish often includes a commitment to responsible fishing practices:

1. Wild-Caught Choices: Pegans who consume fish prioritize wild-caught options, as they are often associated with more sustainable and responsible fishing practices.

2. Supporting Sustainable Seafood: Some Pegans consult resources like the Monterey Bay Aquarium's Seafood Watch program to make informed choices and support sustainable seafood options.

3. Awareness of Overfishing:

Pegans are often educated about the risks of overfishing and the importance of choosing seafood species that are not overexploited.

4. Marine Conservation:

Pegans may also support marine conservation organizations and initiatives working to protect oceans and fish populations.

Peganism Beyond the Plate

Peganism is more than just a dietary choice; it's a way of life that extends beyond the plate:

1. Conscious Consumerism:

Pegans are often conscious

consumers who consider the impact of their choices, not only on their health but also on the planet and society.

2. Environmental Stewardship: Peganism often includes a commitment to environmental stewardship, whether through reduced meat consumption, support for sustainable agriculture, or minimizing food waste.

3. Advocacy: Some Pegans are passionate advocates for ethical and sustainable food systems, using their dietary choices as a platform for promoting positive change.

4. Community Engagement: Many Pegans engage with their communities to raise awareness about responsible food choices and share knowledge about ethical and sustainable eating.

In Conclusion

Chapter 6 has illuminated the ethical and sustainable aspects of the Pegan diet, showing how it goes beyond personal health to address broader issues of animal welfare, environmental sustainability, and responsible food choices. By embracing the Pegan diet, you not only nourish your body but also contribute to a more compassionate, ethical, and sustainable food system.

As you continue reading this book, you'll explore practical aspects of Peganism, from recipes to meal planning strategies. You'll also gain a deeper understanding of how the Pegan diet can positively influence your well-being and the world around you. So, get ready to savor the flavors and embrace the ethical and sustainable dimensions of the Pegan way of eating.

CHAPTER 7

Pegan Recipes and Meal Plans

Welcome to Chapter 7, where we dive into the delicious world of Pegan cuisine. This chapter is all about putting the Pegan diet principles into action with practical recipes and meal plans. We'll explore flavorful Pegan dishes, provide meal planning guidance, and inspire you to create a diverse and satisfying Pegan menu. So, let's embark on a culinary adventure that combines health, taste, and sustainability.

Pegan Recipes: A Fusion of Flavor and Health

The Pegan diet is far from bland or restrictive. It's a vibrant fusion of flavors that celebrates the abundance of plant-based foods and the versatility of high-quality proteins. Let's explore some mouthwatering Pegan recipes that showcase the best of both worlds:

1. Pegan-Style Buddha Bowl

Ingredients:

- 1 cup cooked quinoa

- 1 cup roasted sweet potato cubes
- 1 cup sautéed kale or spinach
- 1/2 cup chickpeas, roasted with spices
- 1/4 cup sliced avocado
- 2 tablespoons tahini dressing
- 1 tablespoon pumpkin seeds

Instructions:

1. Assemble cooked quinoa as the base of your bowl.
2. Top with roasted sweet potato cubes for natural sweetness and roasted chickpeas for protein and crunch.

3. Sauté kale or spinach until wilted and place it on the side.

4. Add sliced avocado for creaminess and healthy fats.

5. Drizzle with tahini dressing for extra flavor and finish with pumpkin seeds for a touch of crunch.

2. Pegan-Style Zucchini Noodles with Pesto

Ingredients:

- 2 medium zucchinis, spiralized into noodles
- 1 cup cherry tomatoes, halved

- 1/2 cup basil leaves
- 1/4 cup pine nuts
- 1/4 cup extra-virgin olive oil
- 1/4 cup nutritional yeast
- 2 cloves garlic
- Salt and pepper to taste
- Optional: grilled chicken or tofu for added protein

Instructions:

1. In a food processor, combine basil, pine nuts, olive oil, nutritional yeast, garlic, salt, and pepper. Blend until you have a smooth pesto sauce.

2. In a large skillet, sauté zucchini noodles until slightly tender.

3. Add halved cherry tomatoes and stir for a couple of minutes.

4. Toss the zucchini and tomatoes with the pesto sauce until well coated.

5. If desired, add grilled chicken or tofu for extra protein.

3. Pegan-Style Lentil and Vegetable Soup

Ingredients:

- 1 cup green or brown lentils, rinsed
- 1 onion, diced
- 2 carrots, diced

- 2 celery stalks, diced
- 2 cloves garlic, minced
- 1 can (14 oz) diced tomatoes
- 6 cups vegetable broth
- 1 teaspoon cumin
- 1 teaspoon turmeric
- Salt and pepper to taste
- Chopped fresh parsley for garnish

Instructions:

1. In a large pot, sauté the diced onion, carrots, celery, and garlic until softened.
2. Add lentils, diced tomatoes, vegetable broth, cumin, turmeric, salt, and pepper. Bring to a boil.

3. Reduce heat and let the soup simmer for about 30-40 minutes or until lentils are tender.

4. Serve hot, garnished with chopped fresh parsley.

Meal Planning for Pegans

Effective meal planning is the key to successfully adopting the Pegan diet. It helps you stay on track, reduce food waste, and ensure you have balanced meals throughout the week. Here are some meal planning tips for Pegans:

1. Set Aside Planning Time: Dedicate a specific time each week to plan your meals. This can be as simple as sitting down with a notebook and your favorite Pegan recipe sources.

2. Create a Weekly Menu: Outline what you'd like to eat for breakfast, lunch, and dinner each day of the week. Include snacks if needed.

3. Consider Leftovers: Plan for leftovers when possible. Cook larger batches of soups, stews, or roasted vegetables that you can repurpose into future meals.

4. Keep a Balanced Pegan Plate in Mind: Ensure your

meals follow the Pegan Plate principle of 50% vegetables, 25% lean protein, and 25% healthy fats and complex carbohydrates.

5. Make a Shopping List: Based on your menu, create a shopping list of ingredients you'll need. Stick to your list to avoid impulse purchases.

6. Prep Ahead: Spend some time prepping ingredients over the weekend. Wash and chop vegetables, marinate proteins, and cook grains. This can save you time during the week.

7. Stay Adaptable: Be flexible with your meal plan. If you don't feel like what you initially planned for dinner, swap it with another meal from your plan.

8. Embrace Variety: Explore new recipes and ingredients to keep your meals exciting. The Pegan diet offers a wide range of flavors and options.

Sample Pegan Meal Plans

To provide you with a practical sense of how to structure your meals, here are two sample Pegan meal plans for a day:

Pegan Meal Plan 1:

Breakfast: Pegan-Style Smoothie

- Ingredients: Spinach, frozen berries, almond butter, almond milk, protein powder
- Instructions: Blend all ingredients until smooth.

Lunch: Pegan-Style Quinoa Salad

- Ingredients: Cooked quinoa, mixed greens, cherry tomatoes, cucumber, red onion, grilled chicken (optional), olive oil and lemon juice dressing

- Instructions: Toss all ingredients together and drizzle with dressing.

Snack: Carrot and Celery Sticks with Hummus

Dinner: Pegan-Style Stuffed Bell Peppers

- Ingredients: Bell peppers, cooked quinoa, black beans, corn, diced tomatoes, spices
- Instructions: Mix cooked quinoa, black beans, corn, diced tomatoes, and spices. Stuff the mixture into bell peppers and bake until peppers are tender.

Pegan Meal Plan 2:

Breakfast: Greek Yogurt with Berries and Almonds

- Ingredients: Greek yogurt, mixed berries, sliced almonds, honey (optional)
- Instructions: Top yogurt with berries, almonds, and honey.

Lunch: Pegan-Style Lentil Soup

- Ingredients: Homemade lentil soup (prepared ahead)
- Instructions: Reheat the soup and enjoy.

Snack: Sliced Avocado with Cherry Tomatoes

Dinner: Pegan-Style Stir-Fried Tofu and Vegetables

- Ingredients: Cubed tofu, broccoli florets, bell peppers, snap peas, ginger-soy sauce
- Instructions: Stir-fry tofu and vegetables in a pan with ginger-soy sauce until cooked through. Serve over brown rice.

In Conclusion

Chapter 7 has delved into the world of Pegan recipes and meal planning, offering you a taste of the flavorful and health-conscious dishes that this dietary approach has to offer. From vibrant Buddha bowls to comforting lentil soup, Pegans enjoy a diverse and satisfying menu that aligns with their values of health, sustainability, and ethical eating.

As you continue reading this book, you'll further explore the benefits and practical aspects of the Pegan diet. You'll also gain insights into the ethical and sustainable dimensions of Peganism, including its positive impact on animal welfare and the environment. So, get ready to savor the flavors and embark on your own culinary journey with the Pegan diet as your guide.

CHAPTER 8

Embracing the Pegan Lifestyle

Welcome to the final chapter of our exploration into the Pegan diet. Chapter 8 goes beyond the plate, focusing on the broader Pegan lifestyle. In this chapter, we'll delve into mindful eating practices, the importance of physical activity, and strategies for long-term success with the Pegan diet. We'll also discuss how to maintain balance and make the

Pegan lifestyle work for you in the real world.

The Mindful Pegan Eater

Mindful eating is an essential aspect of the Pegan lifestyle. It encourages a deeper connection with food, promotes awareness of eating habits, and fosters a more positive relationship with what you consume. Here are some mindful eating practices that align with the Pegan way of life:

1. Eat with Awareness: Pay attention to your food, savoring each bite. Avoid eating in front of screens or while distracted. This allows you to fully experience the flavors and textures of your meals.

2. Listen to Your Body: Tune in to your body's hunger and fullness cues. Eat when you're hungry and stop when you're satisfied, not overly full.

3. Enjoy the Process: Engage in the process of cooking and preparing your meals. Cooking can be a therapeutic and satisfying activity that deepens your connection to food.

4. Savor the Flavors: Notice the flavors in your food. Explore the intricate tastes of different vegetables, herbs, and spices. The Pegan diet offers a rich tapestry of flavors to enjoy.

5. Be Grateful: Cultivate gratitude for the food on your plate and the journey it took to reach you. Recognize the effort of farmers, producers, and all those involved in the food supply chain.

6. Minimize Emotional Eating: Avoid using food as a coping mechanism for stress, boredom, or other emotions. Instead, find healthier ways to address emotional needs, such as mindfulness practices or physical activity.

Physical Activity and the Pegan Lifestyle

Physical activity is a crucial component of the Pegan lifestyle. Regular exercise not only supports overall health but also complements the dietary principles of the Pegan diet. Here's how physical activity aligns with Peganism:

1. Energy Balance: Engaging in physical activity helps maintain a healthy energy balance, especially when combined with the nutrient-dense Pegan diet. This balance is essential for weight management.

2. Cardiovascular Health: Exercise contributes to heart health, which is further enhanced by the heart-healthy components of the Pegan diet, such as omega-3 fatty acids from fish and healthy fats from avocado and nuts.

3. Muscle Health: Physical activity, including resistance training, supports muscle health. This is important for overall strength and vitality.

4. Stress Reduction: Exercise is a natural stress reliever. Stress management is a vital part of the Pegan lifestyle, as chronic stress can negatively impact health.

5. Mind-Body Connection: Certain forms of exercise, such as yoga or tai chi, promote a strong mind-body connection, aligning with the mindfulness aspects of Peganism.

6. Sustainability: Walking, cycling, or using public transportation instead of driving can align with Pegan principles by reducing your carbon footprint.

Sustainable Practices in the Pegan Lifestyle

Sustainability is a core value of the Pegan lifestyle, extending beyond the dietary choices to encompass various aspects of daily life. Here are some sustainable practices that Pegans often embrace:

1. Sustainable Transportation: Whenever possible, choose eco-friendly transportation options such as walking, biking, carpooling, or using public transit. Reducing the use of personal vehicles aligns with sustainability goals.

2. Minimalism: Many Pegans practice minimalism by focusing on essential possessions and reducing waste. This lifestyle choice promotes sustainability by consuming fewer resources.

3. Eco-Friendly Choices: Opt for eco-friendly products in your daily life, from household cleaning supplies to personal care items. These choices help reduce your environmental impact.

4. Gardening: Some Pegans embrace gardening, growing their own vegetables and herbs. This not only provides fresh, organic produce but also connects them with the source of their food.

5. Conscious Consumerism: Pegans are conscious consumers who research and support companies and products that align with their values of sustainability, ethical production, and environmental responsibility.

Strategies for Long-Term Pegan Success

Sustainability in the Pegan lifestyle also means maintaining this way of life for the long term. Here are some strategies to ensure your success as a Pegan:

1. Gradual Transition: If the Pegan diet is a significant departure from your current eating habits, consider transitioning gradually. Start by incorporating Pegan meals and progressively expand your Pegan choices.

2. Build a Support Network: Connect with others who share your Pegan journey. Join online communities, attend Pegan-focused events, or find a Pegan buddy for mutual encouragement.

3. Experiment and Adapt: The Pegan diet is flexible, allowing you to adapt it to your preferences and needs. Experiment with different recipes and approaches until you find what works best for you.

4. Plan and Prepare: Effective meal planning and preparation can save time and ensure you have Pegan-friendly options readily available.

5. Be Mindful of Nutrients: Pay attention to your nutrient intake, especially if you have specific dietary requirements or restrictions. Consult with a healthcare professional if needed.

6. Stay Informed: Stay up to date with the latest research and developments in the Pegan field. This knowledge can help you make informed choices.

7. Practice Self-Compassion: Be gentle with yourself on your

Pegan journey. If you slip up or make less-than-ideal choices, remember that it's all part of the learning process.

8. Reflect and Realign: Periodically reflect on your Pegan journey and realign with your goals and values. This practice ensures that your Pegan lifestyle remains meaningful and sustainable.

Balancing the Pegan Lifestyle in the Real World

Balancing the Pegan lifestyle in the real world can sometimes present challenges. Social gatherings, travel, or simply busy schedules can test your commitment to the Pegan way of life. Here are some tips for navigating these situations:

1. Plan Ahead: When attending social events or traveling, plan your Pegan meals or snacks in advance. This preparation ensures you have Pegan-friendly options available.

2. Communicate Your Needs: Don't hesitate to communicate your dietary preferences and needs to hosts or restaurants. Many establishments are accommodating and willing to provide Pegan options.

3. Flexibility: In situations where Pegan options are limited, be flexible. Choose the best available options while keeping the Pegan principles in mind as much as possible.

4. Home Cooking: Whenever possible, prepare meals at home. This gives you full control over the ingredients and allows you to create delicious Pegan dishes.

5. Pegan Travel Tips: When traveling, research restaurants and markets in advance. Carry Pegan-friendly snacks for convenience.

6. Educate Others: Share your knowledge about the Pegan diet with friends and family. This can lead to more accommodating and understanding environments.

Closing Thoughts

Chapter 8 has expanded our understanding of the Pegan lifestyle, emphasizing the importance of mindful eating, physical activity, sustainability, and long-term success. Embracing the Pegan way of life goes beyond dietary choices; it's a holistic approach to health and well-being that aligns with ethical and environmental values.

As you conclude your journey through this book, remember that the Pegan lifestyle is not about perfection but about progress. Each step you take towards mindful, sustainable, and health-conscious choices is a step towards a healthier you and a better world. So, continue savoring the flavors, nurturing your body, and making choices that align with your values as you embrace the Pegan lifestyle.

CONCLUSION

In conclusion, the Pegan diet is a fascinating and holistic dietary approach that blends the best of both paleo and vegan philosophies. This dietary framework prioritizes whole, nutrient-dense foods, primarily vegetables, fruits, nuts, seeds, and high-quality proteins. It encourages the avoidance of processed foods, refined sugars, and unhealthy fats, making it a health-conscious choice for those looking to improve their well-being.

Throughout this book, we've explored the various aspects of the Pegan diet, from its foundational principles to its health benefits, ethical considerations, and practical implementation. We've learned about its positive impact on heart health, weight management, blood sugar control, gut health, and reduced inflammation. We've also delved into how the Pegan diet promotes ethical eating by supporting animal welfare and environmental sustainability.

Furthermore, we've uncovered the practical side of the Pegan lifestyle, including delicious recipes, meal planning strategies, and tips for long-term success. We've emphasized the importance of mindful eating, physical activity, and sustainability in the Pegan way of life, all of which contribute to a holistic approach to health.

Ultimately, the Pegan diet is more than a dietary regimen; it's a philosophy that encourages conscious and responsible choices in food consumption. It offers a path to better health, ethical eating, and environmental stewardship. By embracing the

Pegan lifestyle, you can embark on a journey toward optimal well-being for yourself and contribute to a healthier, more compassionate, and sustainable world.

As you continue your exploration of the Pegan diet and lifestyle, remember that it's essential to adapt it to your individual needs and preferences. Whether you choose to incorporate Pegan principles gradually or fully commit to this way of life, the key is to find a balance that works for you and aligns with your values. So, savor the flavors, embrace mindfulness, stay active, and make choices that promote your health, the welfare of animals, and the well-being of our planet.